# AGING IN PLACE:

## HOW TO PROTECT YOUR INDEPENDENCE FOR THE REST OF YOUR LIFE

LANORE DIXON, COTA

✳ Created with Vellum

# INTRODUCTION

## WHO THIS BOOK IS FOR

You may have picked up this book because a family member or loved one is beginning to struggle in their current environment; perhaps Mom's vision has decreased or her balance hasn't returned after that last fall; maybe Dad just doesn't seem to recognize that he's not as strong as he once was and is starting to have minor injuries and falls.

If these situations sound familiar, this book can help you. More importantly, if you recognize that in a few years you may be in the same situation as your elder loved ones, this book was written especially for you.

Bravo for your proactive approach to aging in place! Preparation and foresight are key to protecting your independence. The practical solutions and strategies in this book will help you address and predict safety issues in the home, before your function becomes compromised. Now is the perfect time to start.

WHY I WROTE THIS BOOK

I work in the field of geriatric home health. Each day I go into the field to teach patients and their family members how to navigate the new challenges of their health with strategies and home adaptations to keep them safe while they regain their function. Every situation, every home, and every individual is different. But the comment I hear most often is "If I had known this was going to happen, I would have..." Sometimes the comment ends with what the client would not have done rather than with what they would have done.

While it's certainly true that being able to imagine our future may help us plan for it, most of us don't have that skill. I can't tell you or your loved ones what kind of ailments or deficits in physical strength might befall you. But my experience with aging in place can help you prepare yourself, your family, and your environment to protect and support your safety and health so that you can stay in your own home longer.

If you knew, for example, that not being able to get on and off the toilet would someday send you to a nursing facility, I doubt you'd have any difficulty with the idea of installing grab bars or a tall toilet if it meant you could remain in your own home. If you knew that one day you'd slide off the bed and break a hip because your balance and strength no longer allowed you to remain stable while perched on the edge of your tall bed, I bet you'd have no problem making sure the height of your bed was more suited to you. We would change so many things if only we knew they would one day deliver us an experience that could dramatically compromise our independence.

I know how important it is to me to maintain my independence. I've known many families who would do anything to be able to keep their parents or grandparents at home and out of the nursing facility, if only they could assure their safety.

This book provides practical solutions, adaptations, and strategies to live safely and comfortably in your own home, regardless of your age. I'll also give you tools so you can be proactive in your approach to home safety and learn to predict and prevent unsafe situations and accidents. By following these strategies, you can improve safety to protect both you and your loved one's personal independence for years to come.

As you read, please know that I'm not suggesting that you immediately buy all the equipment and gadgets mentioned in this book. But if you start to think about your independence in the proactive manner encouraged here, you may well avoid regrets later. Good intentions aside, most of us can't easily afford home alterations after retirement, especially while paying for medical treatment. If you think about these situations now, you can plan for them before you actively need them and stay healthy, happy, and independent in the comfort of your own home for as long as you choose.

Lanore Dixon, COTA
   2020

# BECOMING SAFETY AWARE

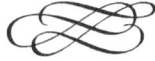

My grandson is approaching three years old. He's full of energy, discovering everything the world has to offer. He is afraid of dolls that talk but is completely fearless of the head injury he could sustain from jumping up and down on the bed. At his age, he needs the wisdom of parents around him to help him stay safe. When he is 16 and takes the wheel of a car, he will have a different level of fearlessness and safety awareness.

. . .

Because our safety awareness changes throughout development, we need different strategies at each level. After we reach adulthood we typically have decades of smooth sailing in safety awareness. But as our physical body changes and our function declines, so does our awareness of our safety.

Addressing changes in our functional decline makes us safer as we age. Several conditions can contribute to a decline in safety awareness as we age. Neurological conditions such as Parkinson's disease, Alzheimer's disease, and other types of dementia, as well as, strokes, brain injuries, and urinary tract infections can have a profound effect on safety awareness. Functional decline in general seems to result in decreased safety awareness.

What can be done about decreased safety awareness as we age? Being proactive and committed to safety now will help us recognize and avoid mental attitudes that compromise our safety and contribute to injuries and falls as we age.

This book offers practical suggestions for environmental changes that you can adopt immediately. But even if you were to rush out this very moment to purchase and install every piece of equipment and make every structural change I suggest in this book, none of that will ensure your safety as much as a proactive mindset toward safety. Even if you ignore everything else in this book, you can better protect your future health if you begin now to adopt habits that prioritize safety in everything you do, particularly at home. Habits take time to form and the sooner you begin them, the better they will serve you when your mindset may wrongly convince you that you are unbreakable.

## Developing Safe Habits and Attitudes

As you read through this book and make the environmental changes suggested, you can also practice the behavioral changes I suggest. If you consistently use these new behaviors, you'll see benefits for years to come. They'll become your natural way of performing tasks, which are dictated more by neuro pathways, often referred to as "muscle memory", than by conscious awareness.

People tend to perform tasks by habit: we get out of bed on the same side, in the same way each day. We brush our teeth, step into the shower, and dress using the same postures and methods every day. We usually only step outside these routine ways of getting things done when our health or the structure of our home forces us.

If you've been standing up to put on your pants your entire life, for example, it's unlikely you'll make a decision at age eighty to sit down to dress, especially if someone else tells you to.

.  .  .

When loved ones or health care professionals lecture on safety and try to change the way you've done things your whole life, you may resent it. You can avoid that annoyance if you commit to learning and adopting the safest behaviors and strategies now. (And yes, it's a good idea to sit down while dressing!) By the time you get to that age when you once again think you're bulletproof, your habits will truly be safe and you'll be better prepared to avoid injury and falls as you age.

As we move toward our sixties, seventies, eighties, and even nineties, educating ourselves about common changes in physical and mental status, preparing our homes, and developing new habits and routines can protect our independence and make our golden years truly golden instead of riddled with increased medical bills, pain, and debilitating injury.

CULTIVATING A PROACTIVE ATTITUDE TOWARD SAFETY

As you develop your commitment to keeping your independence as you age, you can cultivate an even deeper safety awareness by sharing this information with others. By developing and sharing your own passion for safety, you can help friends and loved ones live safer, healthier lives.

Our population is aging. According to the U.S. Census Bureau, by 2035 there will be more adults over the age of 65 than there will be children in this country. More and more people are reaching retirement age and want to continue living healthy, vibrant, and active lives. Help them to do that by making safety awareness a hot topic. Your attitude toward safety will become infectious when you open discussions and share information at Sunday School, golf, bridge club, the senior center, the gym, dance class, or any place you interact with others. By sharing safety information with others, you'll be even more aware and focused on it yourself, relieving your family of worry for your safety.

# FALL PREVENTION AND SAFETY

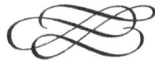

Falls account for a huge percentage of injury, decreased function, and mobility problems as we age.

Fall risk may increase as we age due to losses in:

- Strength
- Balance
- Vision
- Hearing and vestibular function
- Bone density

- Tactile sensory functions
- Safety awareness

Maintaining a healthy diet, adequate hydration, and participating in strength and balance training programs can help prevent falls. In addition, behavioral and environmental adaptations can prepare us for the decline in function that often lead to falls.

After an illness or injury such as a fall, you might find that it's necessary to incorporate environmental adaptations such as ramps at entryways and wider doorways throughout the home. But behavioral changes may the best preventative of disability as we age.

DENIAL AND RESISTANCE TO SAFETY

No one wants to fall. But people can often become convinced, even after having a fall, that their desire to avoid falls will prevent them from experiencing one. Unfortunately, gravity doesn't work that way. Falls happen for a reason and it's seldom that someone invites them consciously.

Many falls are predictable based on habits and behavior. People are usually skeptical when I tell them that therapists know beforehand who is going to fall. No, we don't have psychic powers. But we *do* have plenty of experience in observing habits and attitudes toward safety.

A well-meaning older gentleman once told me I should be teaching patients *how* to fall safely, instead of how to avoid falls. He told me about a man he saw on a talk show who taught nursing homes residents the "right way" to fall to decrease injury.

Even if the man's face hadn't been bruised from one of his own recent falls, I would've deemed him a fall risk based on his attitude toward safety and fall prevention. He didn't believe falls could be avoided and felt it was a waste of time to try.

Most people don't have such glaring evidence of poor safety awareness and fall risk, but we all have the ability to fool ourselves sometimes. You may have observed similar stubbornness and resistance to change in others, but ask yourself where you may be resistant to changing your habits or adopting strategies that could prevent a fall in your own life. If you detect resistance now, be aware that as you age that same resistance can become a barrier to your safety and can compromise your independence.

Some individuals who once had very keen safety awareness actually develop poor safety awareness as they encounter decreased mobility and function in aging. Sometimes when their independence, strength, and health is challenged, they'll resist using assistive devices such as canes or walkers in an effort to become stronger and less dependent on such devices. But abandoning their walker does not make them stronger; it just makes them less safe. In fact, the added weight on upper extremities when using a walker actually increases upper body strength.

Sometimes these individuals are in denial and simply don't want to believe they need a walker or cane. Other times they honestly forget to use it because they aren't used to it. They might leave a walker parked outside the bathroom because it doesn't fit through the door. When they finish in the bathroom, they go back to what they were doing, leaving the walker parked where they left it. Often, they won't even bother taking it to the bathroom at all. It's just a few steps, they reason. And when asked, these individuals will insist they always have their assistive devices with them.

·  ·  ·

I visited a lady recovering from hip surgery who parked one walker beside her chair, another in front of her chair, and another near the front door. When she made her way to the front door, she touched each of these walkers positioned along her path. To her mind, if she merely touched each walker on her way to the door, she was "using" the walker. I told her if she lost her balance while making this trek, she would find the carefully positioned walkers of no use at all and she would fall. But until she actually fell, no one could convince her she was being unsafe.

This is an example of how a poor attitude and lack of compliance can sabotage safety in the home. This woman had changed her environment, placing walkers everywhere, providing herself an abundance of visual cues to remind herself to use them. But her attitude worked against her safety. In order to prevent falls, you must use strategies that work, not just those you find convenient.

. . .

## COMPLIANCE AND COMMITMENT TO SAFETY

When seat belts became required equipment in cars in 1968, the number of fatalities didn't drop significantly. But the effectiveness of compliance with seatbelt use is obvious when you compare states that adopted mandatory seat belt use laws to those that did not. Fatalities in motor vehicle accidents dropped by as much as 23% in states with mandatory seat belt use laws.

In other words, all the best equipment in the world won't help keep you safe if you don't use it correctly and consistently. And you won't use it consistently if you aren't committed to your safety 100% of the time.

Once your commitment to safety becomes part of who you are, everything gets simpler. The choices you'll make, while not always the most convenient ones, are almost always the safer ones. And before you know it, the safer choice becomes so natural you won't even have to think about it. You'll develop neuro pathways, or muscle memory, for performing tasks safely.

Developing neuro pathways for safety becomes even more important with a dementia diagnosis. It's much easier to keep individuals with dementia safe if they have ingrained safe habits. The muscle memory that comes from embracing safe practices early on can become deeply ingrained in behavior, keeping the individual safe long after the mind becomes unreliable to make safe choices.

FALL PREVENTION THROUGHOUT THE HOME

Some places in the home obviously present increased safety concerns and a higher risk of falls. Showers, steps, or a cluttered environment often come to mind when we think about fall prevention. But many falls happen in seemingly unlikely places and circumstances: retrieving items from the closet, getting out of bed, preparing meals in the kitchen. Many falls are often associated with particular kinds of movement. In the following sections, I'll discuss the risk factors for falls in each room in the home, how these falls occur, how particular types of movements and postures contribute to them, and what can be done to address these problems. While these risks may seem minimal and even trivial to an able-bodied person, the complications of aging or illness make them very real and dangerous risks.

## FALL PREVENTION IN THE BEDROOM

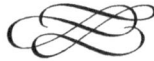

*L*et's take one of the most common fall situations: getting in and out of bed. The problems often arise with the height of the bed and with mattress pads that overhang the mattress. An overhanging mattress pad is just like sitting on a slide: it will carry you right from the edge of the bed to the floor in no time. Make sure mattress pads and mattresses are secure. You can buy non-slip mattress grip pads, similar to non-slip rug pads, to place under mattress pads and mattresses to prevent them from sliding.

· · ·

Many beds are not the ideal height for optimal safety. But it's hard to convince people of this since they've had the same beds for years and have had no problems. And while it may be true that they've had no problems in all those years, as they age and face more problems that occur with declining strength or balance, the height of the bed becomes an increasing risk.

Ideally, when you sit on the bed, your knees will be at a 90-degree angle and your feet will be flat on the floor. If the bed is too tall, buttocks are angled above the knees and toes are on the floor with the heel above the floor. This position may feel perfectly secure, but add in the factors that so typically go with aging or illness, and you've got a formula for a fall.

Sitting edge of the bed like this with only the toes touching the floor, a person can slide off the mattress and onto the floor before they can stop themselves. This risk is even greater if there's an unanchored rug under their feet, or if mobility problems deter their ability to push the hips further back onto the bed.

Many times, people will incur more injuries with this type of fall because they try to stop the fall by grabbing the bedside table, pulling it over on themselves or unsettling the contents on top of it.

REMEDIES

It's not always easy to address the height of the bed. Ideally, the height of the bed should measure about mid-thigh. The risk of sliding out of the bed increases when the bed is any higher. When the bed height is lower than mid-thigh, the buttocks is lower than the knees when in sitting position, making standing more of a struggle.

Some ways you can decrease the height of the bed include removing wheels from bed frames, removing bed frames and placing mattresses on the floor, and removing extra mattresses or pads. While these may not be ideal, they avoid the potential for injuries caused by sliding out of bed onto the floor.

A six-foot-tall man who shares a bed with a five-foot-tall woman may have a problem with the height of the bed, and vice versa. Electric, adjustable beds might seem to solve this problem, but the height of adjustable beds can only be lowered so far. Even the lowest height setting on these beds is too high for some individuals. But there are ways to compensate.

First, bed rails can provide some stability for sitting at the edge of the bed. Typically, a bed rail is anchored under the mattress, near the head of the bed, and allows the individual to push up into standing more easily, especially if the bed is a bit lower than ideal. These are available at medical supply stores and online locations such as Amazon.com.

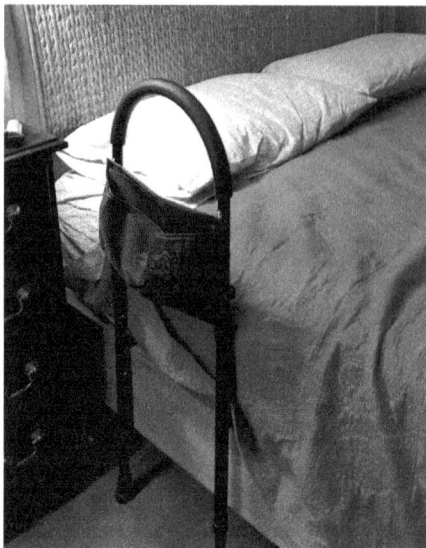

Bed rail

Second, if the person can step up and step down with safety, a low platform, such as an adjustable step aerobics platform can be placed beside the bed to address height problems. These items are available at sporting goods stores, big box stores such as Walmart and Target, and online.

Third, non slip strips near the bedside help to

prevent the individual's feet from sliding when sitting on the edge of the bed.

Further, using proper body mechanics when rising from the edge of the bed helps to prevent falls.

BODY MECHANICS FOR MOVING FROM SITTING TO STANDING

Using the proper body mechanics when transitioning from a sitting to a standing position can help prevent falls and decrease effort required. First, position your feet shoulder-width apart with knees bent and your feet close to the sitting surface. This will make it easier to shift your weight from the buttocks to the feet while providing a wide base of support for stability once you are standing.

Next, position your hands to allow yourself to push up and forward from the sitting surface. If you're sitting at the edge of a bed, your hands should be on the mattress or on the bed rail. If you're sitting in a chair with arms, position your hands on the chair arms. If you sit on a surface with no arms or rails, position your hands on the sitting surface, near each thigh, or put one hand on top of each thigh.

To transition from sitting to standing, shift your upper body forward over your feet to shift your weight from your buttocks to your feet. Then push up and *forward* with your arms and legs from the sitting surface, pushing into a standing position. Pushing forward as well as up from the sitting surface provides forward momentum and decreases the force of gravity during the "lift-off" phase of the movement. Using proper body mechanics also keeps your weight from shifting back into the buttocks and pulling you backwards onto the sitting surface, which also means less wear and tear on the knees.

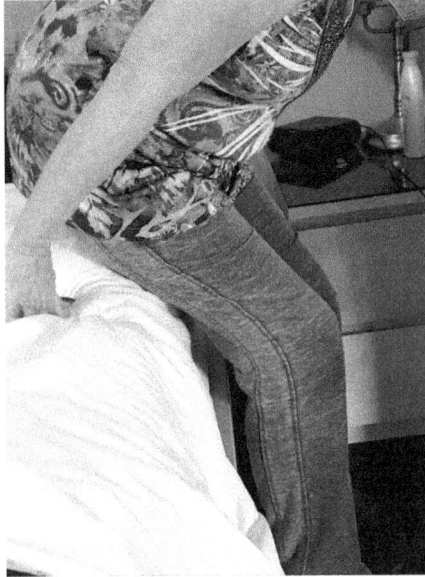

**Forward Weight Shift for Transition to
Standing**

These strategies will help remedy problems
with bed height, but that doesn't mean it's safe
to have a bed that's too tall. In fact, if you adjust the bed height *and* incorporate the above
strategies, you'll decrease fall risk con-
siderably.

# FALL PREVENTION IN THE CLOSET

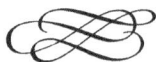

Falls occur in closet areas for a couple of reasons. One, the closet floor is often cluttered with shoes and storage items. Two, people often look upward in the closet, their neck arched backward in extension. This position affects the fluid in their ears, compromising their balance. When we turn our heads in this position, searching for items on upper shelves in the closet, balance is affected even more.

When a person loses their balance in the

closet, they invariably reach for the hanging clothes, grasping frantically for stability and of course, find none. Down they go, often injuring themselves further on boxes and other items stored in the closet.

A simple solution to this type of fall, though not easy, is to clear everything out of the closet that you don't absolutely need on a daily basis.

I sense this suggestion will meet with some resistance because our closets are a favorite place to store all the stuff we don't use every day. Fair enough. But if you use your closet for storage, you should consider keeping the things you use every day in a different location.

For example, I keep my work clothes in my office closet because I get dressed in my office every morning once I finish my morning writing. Other creative solutions people have used have been to hang a small rack on the bathroom door where they place their weekly clothing selections along with one or two pairs of shoes they'll be wearing during the week. This allows them to get dressed as soon as they finish bathing, avoiding the closet altogether.

An acquaintance of mine has a walk-in shower, as well as tub shower in her bathroom. She doesn't use the walk-in shower for bathing, but instead uses it for a closet! She places her shoes on the built-in shower seat and hangs her clothes on a portable clothing rack that stands in the middle of the shower. It's a solution that keeps the bathroom tidy and keeps her safe from tripping over obstacles in her closet.

If you don't have the luxury of having both a shower and a tub in your bathroom, you can use over-the-door hanging rods to hang clothes you'll be using during the week.

Otherwise, cleaning the closet remains an option. Ideally, you'll make sure the equipment in the closet accommodates your needs for optimal safety before you have balance deficits.

The following suggestions can make your closet less of a fall risk:

- Place closet rods between shoulder and waist level to decrease the need to look up.
- Store shoes on shelves above the hanging clothes or on shoe racks mounted on the door to avoid bending and searching for them at floor level.
- Arrange clothing items so in-season clothing and most frequently worn

items are placed near the closet door.

- Store seldom-used items on the top shelves of the closet and not on the floor; better, store them in a different location.
- Use shelves, hooks, and hanging shelves to store handbags, scarves, and other accessories to keep them off the floor;
- Install bright lighting in the closet to light your path.
- Keep a reacher handy to avoid stretching too far for items in the closet.
- Install grab bars in the closet.
- Place a small bench or chair inside walk-in closets or near closet doors to provide a place to rest and to sit while dressing or removing clothes and shoes.

Remember, head movement, especially when

you look up, can compromise balance. Be prepared by holding onto a grab bar. Don't be tempted to hold onto clothing: they will *not* support you! Turning your head from side to side can also increase fall risk; move carefully and with awareness. Also, bending over at the waist can shift your weight forward, outside the base of support of your feet, causing you to topple over. Keeping your body in a neutral position and keeping your weight centered over your feet will help to keep you anchored safely on your feet.

# FALL PREVENTION IN THE KITCHEN

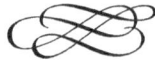

❦

*M*any falls occur in the kitchen. They can happen because of spills, reaching overhead, bending forward too far, moving from one type of flooring to another, and changing directions too quickly, among other reasons.

As mentioned earlier in the discussion about closets, reaching overhead for items in the kitchen cupboard can also disturb balance. You can decrease fall risk from this movement by moving frequently used items to an area between eye level and waist level. This area is prime real estate for the kitchen. Heavy items should also be stored in this zone. This change can also help you avoid injury in your shoulders and back from reaching too high or too low to retrieve heavy items.

When entering a kitchen, you are often transitioning from a carpeted surface to a hard surface. Be aware that changes in surface texture increases fall risk. In addition, kitchen tasks often require a change in direction of 180 degrees, turning from the stove top to the sink, for example. These types of transitional movements are often associated with falls. The brain has to make a raft of calculations to maintain balance when we change direction, and the faster we change, the faster the brain must calculate. Our brains don't always keep up with the speed we're moving while making these transitions, further increasing the fall risk. It is important to slow down and be mindful that your head, shoulders, and feet should all be pointing the same direction to prevent falls when turning around and changing direction.

Wet floors also pose an added fall risk. Spills probably occur in the kitchen more than any other room in the house. Even with non-slip shoes, you can go down in a heartbeat if you slip on spilled liquid on the floor. It's good idea to keep cleaning items handy, such as a mop, throwaway rags, or paper towels to clean up spills as soon as they happen. Using rolling carts or walker trays to clear food or dishes can keep you from carrying more than you safely should.

Like closets, kitchens can be havens for clutter; but as we get older, we typically cook less. Decreased endurance and energy can put a damper on our ambitions for producing elaborate meals. When it becomes obvious that you have less interest in cooking and you'd like to simplify that side of your life, take the opportunity to purge your kitchen just as you would purge your closet of clothes that no longer fit your lifestyle.

Your cooking and kitchen equipment should help you in your current lifestyle, not your lifestyle of 30 years ago. If you don't cook big meals, such as group dinners or feasts for holiday celebrations, get rid of giant serving bowls and pots you no longer use. Give the enormous turkey roaster to your daughter-in-law or to a homeless shelter. Give your grandmother's china to your granddaughter, your pressure-cooker canner to a family member that will make use of it. If you don't have a need for them, there's no need to hang onto things that take up precious space in your home. Make careful decisions about what items you keep in your kitchen and where you will store them.

. . .

Lower cabinets will be safer and much more accessible if they slide out like drawers. But even with the convenience of slide-out cabinets, bending down and lifting kitchen equipment can increase the risk of injury. The heavier the object, the greater the risk. To decrease the risk, store heavier items at waist level and store seldom-used items either in upper or lower cabinets. Bulky, but lightweight items, such as lightweight mixing bowls or bulky, plastic storage containers are best stored in lower cabinets. Use a reacher to retrieve lightweight items stored in lower cabinets and drawers.

Items in upper cabinets are often inaccessible without a step stool. Once your balance becomes an issue, stay away from the step stool and get some help! Do not stand on a chair or other furniture to help you reach items in the upper cabinets. If they are lightweight, retrieve them with a reacher. Make sure you don't try to reach items that are heavier than what your reacher is rated or what your skill level of using it dictates.

Store the items you use the most-- especially if they're heavy--near waist level. This typically means on top of the counter. Some kitchens have deep drawers instead of lower cabinets. These are great for storing larger items, but again, don't store heavy items below the waist--that increases your risk of injury from lifting.

Another huge fall risk comes from having rugs in the kitchen. In fact, rugs pose a safety hazard anywhere in the home. Please remove them!

Ideally, your kitchen floor should be free of anything that can cause you to stub your toe, trip, or catch your walker leg or cane. If you don't do marathon bouts of cooking, you shouldn't need an anti-fatigue mat. Taking frequent rest breaks when you're working in your kitchen is much safer than using a mat. A tall stool that allows you to sit comfortably at your countertop can provide a place to rest as well as a place to perch while you perform kitchen tasks, decreasing fatigue as you work.

# FALL PREVENTION IN LIVING AND DINING AREAS

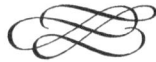

Because we spend so much time in the living and dining areas of our homes, falls often occur there. One of the most common reasons for falls in this area is a cluttered environment. As we get older, not only have we accumulated a lifetime worth of stuff, but each day it gets harder to deal with due to our decreased space and our diminished energy and mobility.

Our living spaces are often cluttered with books, magazines, yesterday's newspapers (okay, last week's newspapers, too) cords for phones, lamps, televisions, electric recliner chairs, etc. We must navigate around large, seldom used pieces of furniture, and rugs. In short, our living spaces can be crowded, messy, and hazardous.

With all of these things to maneuver around, especially if you are on a walker or in a wheelchair, keeping this area tidy becomes an even greater chore. The result is an environment that practically guarantees the mess and the fall risk will continue to grow.

Many people have spent decades trying to downsize their possessions and become more organized. But as we age, the concern about adequate space also becomes a health concern. A messy environment can literally shorten your life with the increased stress and fall risk it poses.

. . .

Of course, we all need to toss out a raft of small items and knick-knacks we've been holding onto, but we also need to consider letting go of larger items that clutter our environments, such as furniture. When we begin to experience decreased balance and mobility, we need even more floor space to navigate safely through our environment. Those large pieces of furniture we've accumulated over our lifetimes can become burdensome.

If there is ever a time to downsize, it's now. Hopefully, you are fortunate enough to merely be approaching the time when your strength and mobility could be affected by age. But it's never too late. I have seen too many people taken by surprise by a turn in their health, finding themselves trapped by their belongings. Too often their family members must take the burden of their personal and household items, dispose of them in the quickest and not the most optimal way. If you are fortunate enough to still enjoy good health and a strong body, now is the time to make decisions about the items in your home that are taking up more than their share of space and may compromise your health and wellness in the future.

When you begin to downsize you will literally feel the burden of all those things being lifted from you, removing a source of stress you didn't realize existed.

When you go through your home searching for items to remove, try to focus on your future and not your past. Don't hold onto a large dining room table just because you have fond memories of family gatherings and holiday meals gathered around it. If you no longer host the holiday meals or the large family gatherings, allow yourself to let go of those furnishings. You have a whole store of memories in your mind; you don't need a mammoth table to remind you of those happy times. And if your home is pleasant and uncluttered, family and friends will enjoy coming to visit you more and you can add to your happy memories.

If you have chairs in your dining areas with rolling casters, either get rid of them or remove the casters, which pose a huge fall risk. You can remove some of the larger pieces of furniture by keeping a limited number of chairs in the living and dining areas. You can buy or trade for folding chairs that you can bring out when you need extra, and save the space the extra seating now occupies. This will also allow you to remove extra end tables and perhaps lamps. Opening up space in your home not only makes your home safer, but it also will make you and everyone in your home feel better. Cramped quarters and clutter are silent stressors, but they take their toll on our health, happiness, and relationships.

As we age, technology continues to move forward, enhancing the convenience of our lives and requiring that we keep our electronic devices charged and powered. Charging stations should be located where they are convenient but do not pose a safety hazard or eyesore. Some charging stations come in attractive cabinets, tables, and other types of furniture. These furnishings must have access to power to charge our devices. Place them near a wall to keep cords out of pathways or use power plates that have been installed in the floor.

Cords and cables should be run along walls and baseboards, well out of traffic areas. Cord and cable management systems are available to accommodate these items attractively and safely. You can find these items at office supply stores, online stores such as Amazon.com and home improvement and electronics stores.

Adequate lighting is also important for safety in living areas. Many living rooms have no overhead lighting and rely only on lamps for light. Having a floor lamp close to the door or the table lamps controlled by the wall switch near the door will eliminate the need to walk through a dark room to turn on a lamp.

Baskets and racks that hold magazines, crafts, and pet toys can be tucked away under tables or in drawers and kept out of pathways. Reachers come in handy to keep these items off the floor eliminating the need to bend or reach too far to pick up items from the floor.

Individuals with mobility problems often set up their immediate environment to accommodate their needs and to require as little walking and standing as possible. A table beside their chair typically holds a lamp, medication bottles, the daily paper, magazines, grooming supplies, lip balm, tissues, remote controllers, a container of water, a reacher, eyeglasses, pens and pencils, hand lotion, the daily mail, telephone, checkbook, postage stamps, snack foods, and other items they might need during the course of the day or night they spend in their chairs. Of course, the table is overflowing and the contents often fall to the floor, as do the blanket and pillow they keep in the chair with them to add to their comfort. It does get uncomfortable when you're stuck in the same place all day, after all. But without a system in place to keep these items organized and confined, the risk of falls steadily increases.

Although the mess may be blossoming in the living room, furniture that is typically used in the bedroom or office may be the best solution to the problem. A small desk, bookcase, chest of drawers, or night table may provide better accessibility to needed items, as well as increase storage capacity, and safety for individuals who spend most of their day confined to a chair.

Suitable furniture for this purpose may already be available in other areas of the home and may only need to be relocated to the living room area. If you have no need at present for repurposing your furniture in this way, consider that you may have a future need and make furniture purchasing decisions with this in mind.

The table beside the chair should contain the most used items and those needed for safety such as the remote control, telephone, drinking water, and tissues. A trash bin can be placed beside the chair to catch junk mail, used tissues, and trash. Blankets and wraps should be draped over the back of the chair when not in use to prevent them from sliding to the floor and creating a fall risk. These simple precautions will make life more convenient and much safer for individuals with compromised mobility.

As mentioned previously, rugs present a fall hazard throughout the home as they can catch on toes or rolling walkers and increase fall risk; If you need to move quickly, a rug can slow you down or completely stop your progress if it catches on your feet, walker, or wheelchair.

It's hard to convince people to get rid of their rugs, especially expensive ones that have been in their lives for a long time. Often, they're used to the rugs so they don't seem like much of a hazard. But once they have to deal with something they're not used to, such as a cane, walker, or wheelchair, suddenly the rug isn't so easy to navigate around. Even then it's difficult for people to part with their rugs.

For example, I cautioned a friend that the rug in her hallway was a fall hazard. It was a nice rug and in good repair, and my friend argued that it had been there for years and they were used to it. Until actual injury occurs, it's hard for most of us to imagine that our familiar surroundings and age-old habits may become risky at some point. But after my friend's husband tripped on the corner of that rug, cracked his skull on a door facing, and broke his hip, she got rid of the rug and began to adopt a more proactive approach to safety in her home. You are an adult and you get to decide what items will stay in your home and which ones need to go. But it's important to understand the risks of your choices. Hopefully all your choices will be safe and you will stay happily in your own home for as long as you choose.

A tidy, well-lit living area, free of excess furniture, rugs and clutter, will provide a safer, more relaxed environment to unwind and enjoy your independence as you age.

# FALL PREVENTION FOR TOILETING

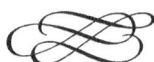

When we consider fall prevention in the bathroom, most people automatically think of falls in the shower or tub. But many falls also occur during toileting. Because fall risk increases in the bathroom, with toileting and bathing carrying task specific risks, I'll cover these areas in separate chapters.

Taller toilets and grab bars go a long way to prevent falls and make the toileting task safer and easier. But one of the most common falls during toileting occurs when people don't line themselves up with the toilet before sitting.

Even when a grab bar is available, poor alignment to the toilet before sitting often results in landing on the floor. Sometimes when people fall while toileting, they become wedged between the wall and the toilet. This is a really tough place to fall. Not only is it painful, as most falls are, it's also embarrassing. Typically, a family member will try to fish you out, but a lot of times you're just stuck there until emergency medical services arrive.

Having such a fall puts you in a truly compromising position. There you are, lying wedged against the cold toilet with your underwear down. Remember, you were going to the bathroom, right? In this situation, emergency services might discreetly cover you, then carefully extract you, check you for cuts and bruises, and maybe encourage you to visit the ER for a more thorough check.

. . .

The easiest way to avoid a fall during toileting is to make sure *both* your legs are touching the toilet before you sit down. In fact, aligning properly to the sitting surface is key to avoiding falls no matter where you're sitting, whether it be the dining room chair, sofa, car seat, bed, or any other place you perch yourself.

If a grab bar is available for toileting, of course, you should use it as needed. Grab bars can be mounted on either or both sides of the toilet, depending on the layout of the room. Grab bars come in horizontal, angled, and swing away types. Grab bars around the toilet are usually mounted horizontally next to the toilet about hip level. These can be straight or angled bars. Angled grab bars provide a horizontal bar to push up on that angles upward about 45 degrees diagonally or 90 degrees vertically to allow the user to pull up into standing position.

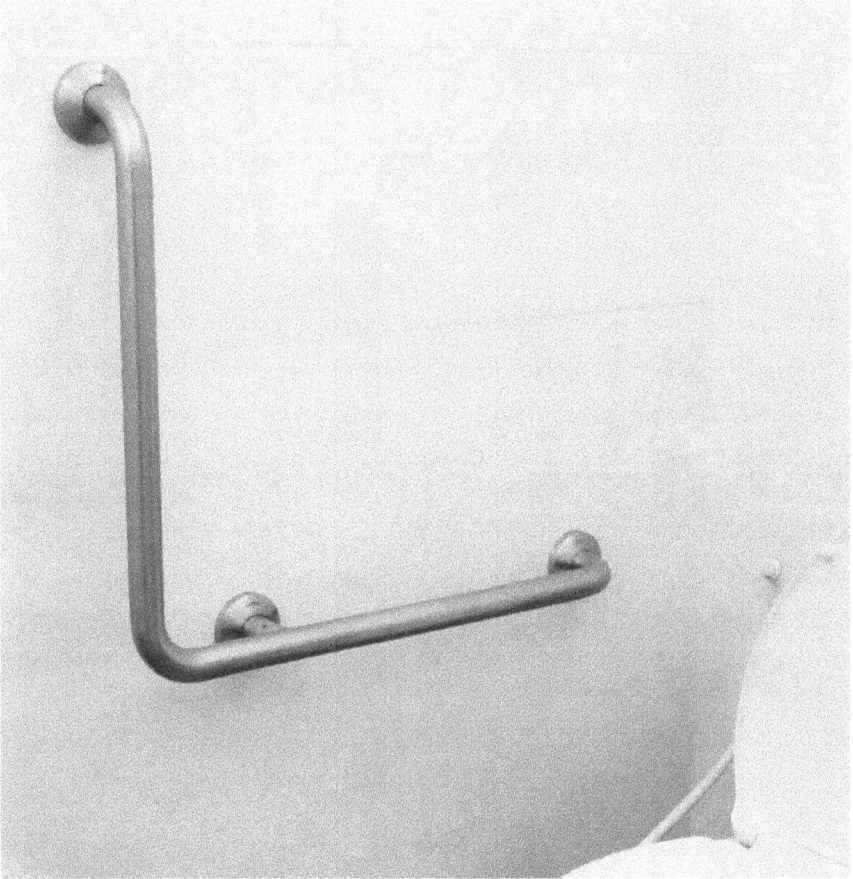

**90-Degree Grab Bar**

Swing away grab bars that fold down from the wall can be mounted to provide support on the side or in front of the toilet. If this type of grab bar is mounted to provide support in front of the user, care must be taken that ample standing room remains between the toilet and the bar to allow forward weight shifting for transitioning from a sitting to a standing position.

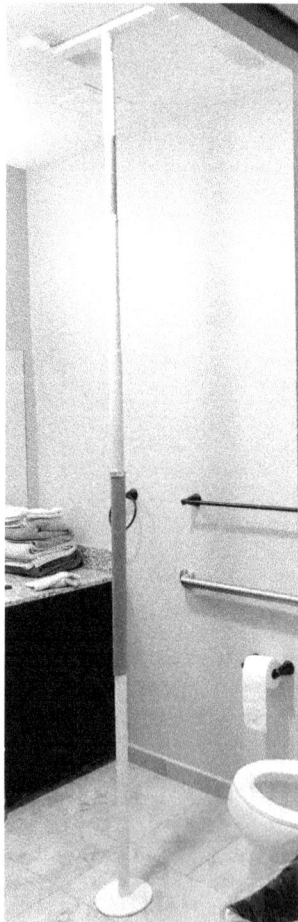

**Vertical Transfer Pole**

Transfer poles, which are vertical poles that extend from floor to ceiling, can be used when a traditional grab bar cannot be mounted on the wall. They can be useful outside shower doors, between showers/tubs and toilets or near a wall that holds a pocket door.

# FALL PREVENTION DURING SHOWERING

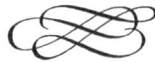

⚜

Increased fall risk is always associated with showering tasks because of the wet, slippery surfaces. Falls can occur while in the shower, stepping in or out of the shower, or over the wall of the tub. When we are able-bodied, these kinds of maneuvers are of little challenge. But even minor mobility problems can make stepping over a tub wall or even a low shower threshold terrifying. Ironically, fall risk increases as fear of falling increases.

. . .

Fortunately, proper precautions and equipment can make shower transfers much safer and less scary. Having adequate room in the bathroom and a shower designed for accessibility can help too. But this book is about using what you have to make it optimally safe for you. This section will discuss strategies and equipment to make the showering task safer. Later, in the section on entryways, we will discuss shower doors.

One of the biggest problems I've seen with the safety in bathrooms is walk-in showers that are too small. I've learned the term "walk-in" is completely relative. If you are an amputee, you will not view a shower with a 6-inch threshold as a "walk-in" shower. Likewise, if you have a diagnosis of Parkinson's disease or diabetes with decreased sensory function in your feet, you may have a real problem safely stepping over that 6-inch threshold.

Generally, the problems with these facilities

can be overcome with the right equipment, such as tub transfer benches. But if a shower is too narrow, or the door is poorly located, even a tub transfer bench may not help.

One solution I've seen for walk-in showers with high thresholds is a cut-out which simply cuts the threshold down to floor level. A flexible rubber lip is installed where the threshold would have been, to keep water confined in the shower. This doesn't always work, however, depending on the construction of your floor, shower, and bathroom. Those types of structural changes are outside the scope of this book, even though you may choose to share these ideas with your contractor to be considered for your particular situation.

A tub transfer bench can work for both a tub or a shower if the tub/shower doorway is accessible and provides enough space for the tub bench. The doorway must also be wide enough to allow you to sit on the bench, then turn around and move your legs inside the tub/shower to face the faucet. One end of the tub transfer bench sits outside the tub, while the other end sits inside the tub. Because you can sit down on the bench while you stand outside the tub, the transfer bench eliminates the need to step over the tub wall. This safety feature will therefore generally serve you better than a shower chair even if your mobility becomes further compromised. I generally advise clients to skip a shower chair altogether and pay the additional ten bucks for the tub transfer bench. Shower benches and chairs are much cheaper than remodeling the tub and shower, of course.

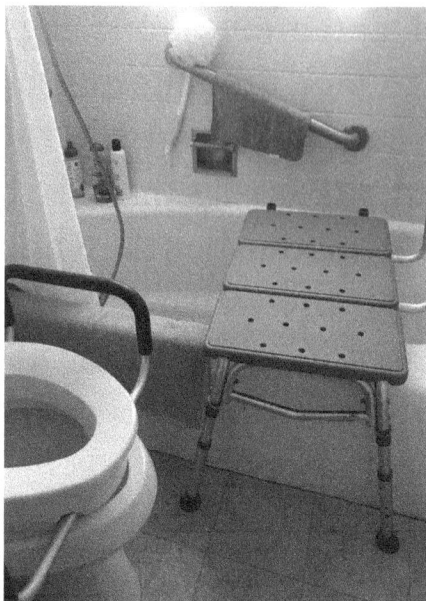

**Tub Transfer Bench**

A common concern about tub transfer benches is that they are too large for many bathrooms. For the most part, this concern is unfounded. These benches extend outside the tub wall 4-6 inches, which is enough to allow the user to safely sit on the bench while standing outside the tub. The bench takes up very little of the usable space in the bathroom. The photo above is an example of how little space is required around the bench to allow safe, easy access to the tub shower. Furthermore, all four legs of the bench are adjustable, providing a level surface to sit on while showering. Tub transfer benches can be used with most tub showers. One exception where they generally will not work is tubs with very tall walls, such as garden tubs.

Another concern about tub transfer benches is that they extend outside the tub, beyond the shower curtain, causing the floor to get wet. The easiest remedy for this is to simply tuck the shower curtain under the user's leg to prevent water from streaming onto the floor. A tidier and more sanitary remedy is to cut a rectangle from the bottom of the shower curtain liner that measures from the front of the bench to the back so that water is directed into the tub and not onto the floor outside the tub.

A hand-held shower head will make the bathing task even safer, allowing you to remain seated for most of the task. The more compromised your mobility, the more important this becomes.

Some showers have built in benches. I am generally not a fan of these for several reasons. Depending on the material they are made of, they are often cold to sit on, they don't drain well and can therefore harbor bacteria. Some shower benches can also be slick, presenting an even greater fall risk.

Often, built-in shower benches are not adjustable in height or position. Benches that are too tall could cause the user to slide off into the floor of the shower. At the same time, standing up from a bench that is too low can be quite difficult. Sometimes built-in shower benches are simply positioned too far from the faucet to safely control the water from sitting position. They can also take up a lot of valuable space. If you are having your "forever" home designed, you would do well to avoid this space hog feature in your shower area unless it is adjustable and positioned optimally for control of the water flow.

If you are buying a home or remodeling, consider your mobility in later years: garden tubs and Jacuzzis in the bath are beautiful and relaxing, but these, as well as standard tubs, may very well become inaccessible to you after age 70 or so and this can be life threatening.

For example, I recently learned of a woman who was forced to stay in her tub for two days because she couldn't get out of it. She had decided to take a bath after her husband left for an out of town trip. She had no trouble getting into the tub, but when it came time to get out, she found she lacked the strength and agility. She struggled until exhausted, but no matter how hard she tried, she couldn't stand up or crawl over the side of the tub. Alone in the house without her phone nearby, she was stuck in the bathtub until her husband returned at the end of the weekend. She spent a miserable weekend, cold, hungry, and alone, able to stay warm only by turning on the hot water every couple of hours.

Fortunately, for those of us who love to take baths, there are safe and convenient alternatives to traditional, garden, and Jacuzzi tubs.

If you are designing your bathroom space, walk-in tubs are an alternative to traditional tubs and garden tubs. Walk-in tubs come with sealed, hinged doors that require the user to stay inside the tub while it fills and empties. Manufacturers claim the units fill and empty quickly so users don't have to sit partially submerged for long. One caveat is cost, as these tubs can run as high as $18,000 per unit installed, a cost that is unrealistic for many senior budgets.

Another alternative to the accessibility problems of traditional tubs is a tub lift. These sit in the bottom of the tub and lower and raise the user into and out of the tub, respectively. The lifts I have seen in use impressed me with their design and ease of use, both for the individual and their caregivers. Weight capacities are rated up to 300 pounds for standard models and up to 500 pounds for bariatric models. Currently, the price of these is between $400 and $600, a more affordable alternative to a walk-in tub.

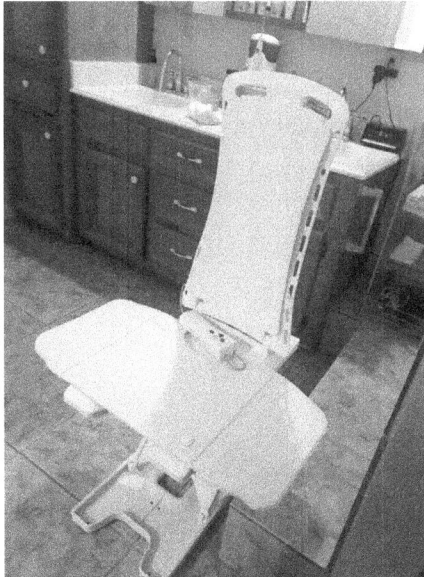

**Tub Lift Chair**

Grab bars in and around the bathing area

also promote safety. A grab bar on the wall outside the shower or tub allows a user to hold on while stepping into the shower. Many people prefer vertically mounted grab bars outside the shower due to limited wall space.

A grab bar inside the shower provides stability when completing the standing part of the showering task; Anchoring systems are now available to allow installation of grab bars without setting them into the studs of the wall, allowing a wide variety of placement options. Textured grab bars are preferable inside the shower to prevent hands from slipping in the wet environment.

Grab bars for the tub/shower are available in every style and configuration imaginable, including shower heads with grab bars and grab bars that clamp to the outside tub wall. In fact, a whole line of grab bar designs and accessories for the shower are available, including shower shelf grab bars and soap dish grab bars.

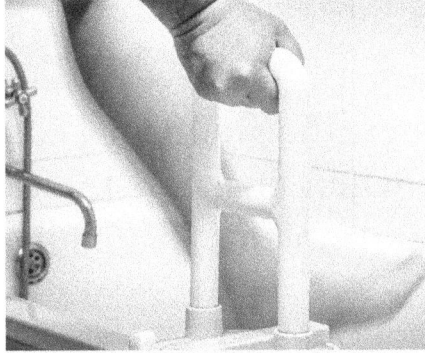

**Tub Clamp Grab Bar**

I generally do not recommend temporary grab bars which come with large suction cups and levers to fasten them onto the surface of the wall. These must be tested for fastness with every single use. This extremely important step is simply too easy to forget and could result in a serious fall. Furthermore, a fall could occur during the process of testing as a proper fastness test would require adequate pressure and exertion on the bar. Far better to consider alternatives to grab bars if one simply cannot be mounted on the wall in the traditional manner.

Transfer poles, as discussed earlier, can be installed between the floor and ceiling outside the shower when inadequate wall space or construction problems prohibit the use of grab bars.

Contrary to what many people believe, bathtub and shower mats can greatly increase the risk of falling during bathing. This information surprises a lot of people because they purchase bath mats to prevent falls. But mats can slide when wet and weight distribution shifts.

Instead of mats, I recommend adhesive floor decals that are available for a few dollars at places like Walmart, Lowe's, Home Depot, etc. The downside of decals is that they will eventually show wear and tear, and collect dirt. Sometimes, they don't stay in place long enough, or they can be very difficult to remove. But even with these problems they are a safer alternative to mats.

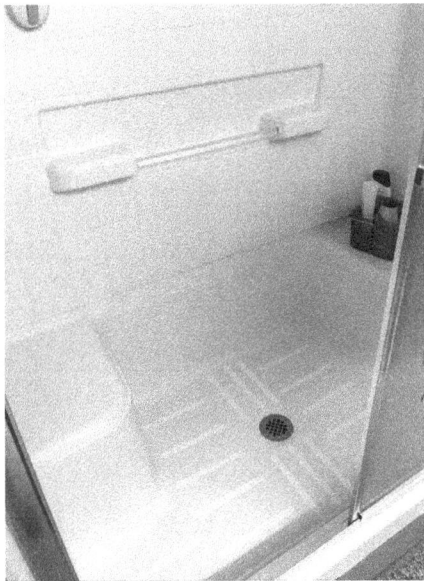

**Non-slip Decals for Shower Floors**

Most of the disadvantages to floor decals can be addressed easily: Clean and rinse the tub/shower floor thoroughly and let it dry for a full 24 hours before applying the decals. By installing decals on a clean, dry, preferably non-porous surface, they'll stay in place much longer.

Important! When shopping for non-slip decals for your bathroom, be very careful to get actual decals with adhesive backing. Don't be fooled by the tub decor items that appear to be decals, but have the dreaded suction cups on the back. These have all the same problems that tub mats have and will slide across the wet tub floor when weight is improperly distributed. Please avoid these at all costs!

If you are building a home, there are some options in non-slip, textured tile for shower floors. Ask your builder about these options; But remember, no matter what surface you decide to install, you'll have to have a system to prevent soap build-up to keep your shower floor safe. If your mobility becomes compromised by age, injury, or surgery, you won't be able to get down on your hands and knees and scrub the shower floor. Who wants to do that anyway? So, before you invest in expensive flooring for your custom-built shower, find out what it's going to take to keep it clean and safe.

Bath rugs are another source of falls in the bathroom area. The floor outside the tub/shower typically is wet after bathing, so a non-slip rug outside the tub or shower makes sense. However, as discussed earlier, rugs pose an increased fall risk throughout the home. To avoid using a rug, some people place towels outside their showers, and sometimes even inside the shower to prevent slipping. But towels can become bunched up, catch on toes, and cause a fall.

For optimal safety, I recommend using a non-slip rug outside the shower *only* during the bathing task. The rug should be removed immediately after the bathing task is finished. No other rugs should be on the floor of the bathroom.

. . .

Remember that as you age, you may have to make a lot of changes to your environment to accommodate changes in function. Also consider that you may very well need a caregiver. When it comes to your bathroom and shower area, the more space you have, the better. In fact, as we age, bathrooms should ideally be big enough to accommodate needed equipment, such as wheelchairs or walkers, *as well as caregivers*.

You may be able to increase the space in your bathroom simply by clearing clutter and furnishings that are not absolutely necessary. Clothes hampers, scales, laundry baskets, freestanding shelves and cabinets, tables, free standing toilet paper dispensers and towel racks, as well as baskets and boxes of items that have been pushed into the bathroom for temporary storage should be cleared from the floor space to allow adequate space for moving about safely in the bathroom.

. . .

If you are building a new home or searching for a home to buy, you want the largest bathroom available. Consider that increasing the size of the bathroom by cutting down the size of your kitchen can be a good trade-off.

Adequate space, proper equipment, and good lighting, including night lights, can greatly improve safety in the bathroom and add years to your independence as you age in place.

# HOME ADAPTATION FOR ACCESSIBILITY

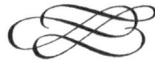

This part of the book takes a look at the accessibility issues that will help you prepare your home for aging in place. Many home adaptations require little or no skill to install and can be added to your home now to help you stay safe and develop safe habits and strategies. As you read, try to think about your own home and how these concepts may help you to address accessibility and safety issues or help you brainstorm solutions of your own.

. . .

Many people automatically think of wide doorways and passageways when they think of aging in place. While these are often necessary for accessibility, there is much more to consider to ensure a home is functional, safe, and appropriate for aging in place.

Try this: take a tour through your home and imagine you're standing inside a box with the same dimensions as wheelchair or rolling walker—usually about 2 x 3 feet. Would you be able to move down the hallway and through all the doorways without touching the walls or door frames? Would it be easy to turn around, go around corners, and back up without bumping into walls? Would you have to perform some serious maneuvering to get through some parts of your home, such as turning sideways to get through doorways with a walker or struggling to make a series of ninety degree turns to get from the hallway to the bathroom or bedroom in a wheelchair?

. . .

If this exercise was awkward and you found it would be difficult to navigate through your home, you might be able to understand some of the frustration of someone in a wheelchair or rolling walker trying to maneuver in such a restricted environment. But even when doorways and thresholds are wide enough, the layout of the home can impede accessibility.

For example, many homes require a 90-degree turn to enter a hallway, then another 90-degree turn into the bathroom or other rooms off the hallway. These angles can create barriers for wheelchair users. This is especially true if the hallway is narrow and there's inadequate room to straighten the wheelchair before turning into the bedroom or bathroom off the hallway.

When my husband and I were looking for a retirement home, this was a problem in many of the houses we saw. A few homeowners had prepared their homes for aging in place: We saw walk-in showers, raised toilets, and entryway ramps; But in most of the homes we saw, access to bathrooms or bedrooms would be difficult in a wheelchair or walker because of the narrow halls and short distances between doorways in the halls. Correcting this type of layout involves major work of widening hall doorways and adding beams, jobs that increase the overall cost of the home, often beyond what the housing budget allows.

These are important issues to consider if you are buying a home. If you already own such a home, you hopefully have time to adapt it for better accessibility before you actually have a need for it.

If you're having a home built, the builder may not have future accessibility needs in mind either. Although the National Association of Home Builders strives to make their products more inclusive of all ability levels, cost factors and a builder's accessible design experience will greatly affect the result.

You are your own best advocate for making your home serve your needs as you age in place. The following sections can help inform your choices and considerations for each area of your home as you prepare for a healthy and safe future.

EXTERIOR ENTRIES

Ideally, an entryway into the home should be flush with the floor inside the door. A threshold of 1/2 inch or less with a bevel lets you easily roll over it in a wheelchair or rolling walker. The doorway should be at least 36 inches wide to allow 32 inches of clear space for entry.

A gently sloping ramp, rather than steps, should lead you to the front door if it is higher than the ground. The American Disabilities

Act (ADA) recommends the slope of ramps be one foot in length for each inch in height for optimal safety and accessibility.

Longer ramps may require landings to allow adequate length for a safe ramp slope. Landings also require a greater ramp width to accommodate for turning radius. Ramps can be built-in or portable, depending on the height of the main entry. Generally, when the entry is more than a foot above the ground, a stationary ramp is more suitable.

Entryways that are closer to ground level have more options available for suitable ramps. Portable and stationary ramps can be made in a variety of styles, custom-made, or prefabricated, with materials from fiberboard to metal.

Prefabricated galvanized ramps without rails or rims can be trimmed for exact fit and rolled up and put away when not in use. These are available online, by mail order, or at big box stores like Home Depot and Lowe's, as well as general hardware stores that can order to specification.

Ramps can be purchased pre-fabricated or built to your specifications. Cost is often a determining factor of the type of ramp available. But you may qualify for one of the many services that provide ramps for those who cannot otherwise afford them. You can find information about community non-profit agencies that provide free or low cost ramp building services at organizations such as United Way, Habitat for Humanity, as well as local veterans organizations and churches. These services are a great help in providing information, materials, or labor for ramp construction to individuals that qualify for help. To quality you must usually have a documented disability. The application process for these agencies can take a while, so planning a safer more accessible entry into your home now can save you from spending time in a nursing facility or rehab center in the future while you wait to have a ramp built.

## INTERIOR DOORS

Hallway, bedroom, and bathroom doors should be wide enough for a wheelchair to roll through. Hallways should be wide enough to turn a wheelchair into the doorways on the hall without getting stuck or using heroic acts to clear the doorway.

Most interior doors in American homes are 30 inches wide. The clear space, or the width of the door opening, is measured from the innermost part of the door, called the door stop, to the edge of the door when the door is open. Measuring this space on a typical 30-inch doorway will leave about 28 inches.

To estimate clear space, measure the width of the door, then subtract approximately 2 inches to arrive at the space available to pass through the doorway. Remember, this is an *estimate*. Exact measurements are required to ensure the wheelchair or rolling walker will actually fit through the doorway.[1]

You can increase the clear space of doorways in several ways. One of the easiest solutions is to remove the door, but that's not always an option. You can also replace the door hinge with an offset or swing-away hinge. These require the wall on the hinged side of the door has clearance to swing fully open. These types of hinges allow an extra 1-1 1/2 inches of clear space, depending on the thickness of the door. This increased width can make a huge difference to someone using assistive devices to access important areas in the home such as bathrooms.[2]

Pocket doors, also called sliding doors, provide another solution to increase the clear space of doorways, but they also have a few drawbacks. For one thing, the wall that re-ceives the sliding door when it opens, or the pocket wall, must be free of any fixture or hardware that may impede the movement of the door into the wall. This means, no grab bars, towel racks, toilet paper holders, elec-trical wiring, or other equipment can be mounted on or inside the wall that receives the door when it slides open. Pocket doors that latch and open with pull tab hardware at the door edge can also be difficult for individ-uals with dexterity or upper limb deficits to access and use. Some pocket doors operate with a spring and only require a bit of pres-sure on the door edge to allow them to pop out of the pocket. This eliminates the need for good manual dexterity required to pull on a tab that allows the user to pull the door out of the pocket. [3]

Barn doors, also called open pocket doors, work in a similar fashion to pocket doors but are fitted on the outside of the doorway. This removes any concern about foregoing grab bars, electrical or other equipment that may be needed on the wall that contains the door. But again, users must be able to pull the door open and shut.[4]

Finally, simply trimming out the door stop in the lower part of the doorway may provide enough space for the wheelchair or walker to pass through, but may compromise privacy.

If none of these solutions are satisfactory, consider widening the doorway. This can be more expensive and time-consuming generally, but in the long term, it may be more aesthetically satisfying. Depending on your situation, it may be more cost effective to hire a professional to make these types of changes.

When analyzing whether to enlarge a doorway, there are a number of things to consider, such as electrical or plumbing features on the wall that shares the doorway. Electrical outlets are easy to move but may require the expertise of an electrician. Plumbing, on the other hand, may not only require a plumber but may likely be cost prohibitive to change at all.

Also, consider the maximum space available in which to enlarge the door opening. It's a good idea to increase the opening wider than you need it. Better to expand larger than necessary now, rather than having to pay for further expansion later when unexpected changes in mobility or function may demand it.

Sometimes structural changes in the home require a more creative approach. For example, if a bathroom door cannot be widened due to the placement of the vanity or bathroom fixtures, another entry point, perhaps from a neighboring bedroom might be possible. In one such redo, the resident used the closet space from the bedroom next door. This enlarged the bathroom by several feet, allowing French doors to be installed on the bathroom entry. It also is important to think carefully about which rooms will be affected by such structural changes and how these changes will affect the flow of movement through the home.

## HARDWARE FOR ACCESSIBILITY

Apart from door width, door hardware can also impede accessibility in the home. The small joints of the hands often become injured, weak, and frail with age. Door levers provide an advantage over doorknobs, requiring less grasp strength. This results in less joint damage and pain and provides better accessibility.

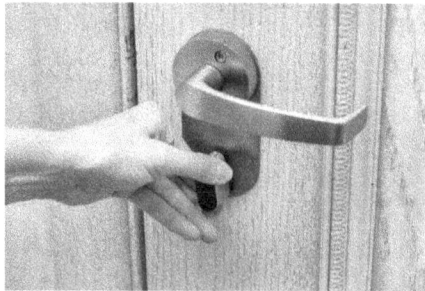

**Lever Door Handle**

Automatic door openers are available for individuals in wheelchairs and magnetic door stops can be used to hold doors open, allowing traffic to pass safely through. These items run about $10 and are available where hardware is sold.

Sometimes the best adaptations are low tech and low expense: A long scarf or sash tied around the door handle will allow the door to be pulled open, or pulled shut once the chair is through it. Heavier doors may require automatic openers.

SHOWER DOORS

Shower doors should be wide enough to accommodate a caregiver and the user. Sliding glass shower doors are a problem for people with mobility issues because they limit the width of access to the shower and the equipment that can be used in bathing tasks. But these can generally be uninstalled easily by removing a few screws in the frame.

Although many beautiful showers are available nowadays, they haven't necessarily been designed with accessibility in mind. For example, I recently saw a gorgeous walk-in shower in a home I visited. It was enormous: 7 x 7 foot with a long, hand-held shower head. The shower bench fit inside with plenty of room to spare for the caregiver. The front of the shower was beautifully glassed on 3 sides. The problem was that the hinged shower door was too narrow to accommodate a walker or wheelchair and allowed no room for a caregiver to walk beside the patient who had very serious mobility problems. The glass walls of the shower could not be modified or equipped with fixtures such as grab bars for safety. Apart from removing the walls, there was little that could be done to adapt the shower for improved safety.

. . .

If you are looking at buying a home, pay close attention to the width and accessibility of the shower, especially the shower door if it has one. Don't allow yourself to be seduced by the aesthetics of the shower or bathroom. The feature you most love could be a problem later on, and a problem you won't want to fix because you love the aesthetics too much.

Safe and accessible entryways, both interior and exterior to the home can add to your years of independence at home. Addressing this issue before it becomes a need is key to aging in place and protecting your independence.

## MULTI-LEVEL HOMES

During the last century multi-level and split floor plans became fashionable. The population in general was younger during those years, so home designers can be forgiven their lack of foresight that has increased the fall risk for baby boomers. What was once so popular has become a home feature that many retiree has paid dearly for, both in medical bills and in remodeling dollars.

A variety of remedies are possible for these homes, depending on the particular design. For multi-storied homes, stair lifts and elevators are options, though expensive ones, for accessing all levels of the home. A more affordable option is to keep living quarters on the ground floor and use upper floors for storage. If these options are not practical, make sure the stairs are equipped with sturdy hand rails, good lighting and non-slip material on stair treads and have a plan so that the majority of your daily activities can be performed on a single floor of the home should it become necessary.

Sunken rooms

Sunken living rooms built in the 1960s and 70s no longer have claim to high fashion in homes. For the aging population, these rooms have increased fall risk and inconvenience in the home. Sometimes the recessed room is shallow enough that a low-cost ramp may be used to make the room safely accessible. But that solution leaves a lot to be desired for aesthetics, as well as safety.

Many homeowners have been able to fill sunken rooms with concrete to bring the floor level up to the other rooms in the home. Other remedies include building a frame to support a new floor the same level as the rest of the home. Depending on the layout and size of the room, it may be necessary to have duct work, electrical outlets, and switches relocated.

## HOME MODIFICATION AND AGING IN PLACE PROFESSIONALS

If you plan on making structural changes in your home, ideally you will have the input of a professional, not only in the building industry but also, in the occupational therapy profession. Many occupational therapists are becoming Certified Aging in Place Specialists (CAPS). You may be able to hire one of these professionals to consult with you or your builder to provide information on the ways that age can affect mobility. These professionals can assist your builder in providing structural solutions to address changes in mobility and function for aging in place.

Make sure you use a professional with good referrals and credentials to work on your home. Finding a qualified, *reputable* contractor can be a challenge. Ask friends and family for recommendations and check your state consumer protection agencies such as the Better Business Bureau for complaints and accreditation before hiring a contractor. Check out https://www.usa.gov/consumer to find consumer protection agencies in your state. Please don't skip this step! A lot of people call themselves contractors but lack the proper skills or the intention to do the job professionally. We've all heard horror stories about money spent on carpentry and other work on the home, only to have the contractor abandon the job with the client's money in their pocket.

Senior citizens are a common target for these individuals. AARP, the senior advocacy organization, has numerous articles educating seniors to protect against such scammers.

To find or verify credentials for contractors who are Certified Aging in Place Specialists, check the National Association of Home Builders website:

https://www.nahb.org/NAHB-Community/Directories/Local-Associations#sort=relevancy

Due diligence is vital to ensure the work will be done professionally, by someone qualified to understand the accessibility needs of the aging population.

. . .

[1] Renda, Marnie, OTR/L, CAPS, ECHM. "Home Modifications: Entrances." Online lecture, MedBridge Education, January 2018. <www.medbridgeeducation.com/course-player/play/7167>

[2] Ibid.

[3] Ibid.

[4] Ibid.

# ADAPTING FOR LOW VISION

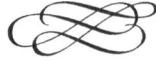

❧

Low vision is a common problem as people age. Macular degeneration, glaucoma, and diabetic retinopathy are common causes of low vision and blindness in adults. Declining ability to see in dim light and decreased color perception also contribute to visual impairment as we age. Low vision can dramatically affect our safety and independence as we age.

Adaptations for low vision in the home can make aging in place safer, more comfortable and convenient. Many of these adaptations are affordable and require no special skills.

LIGHTING

Probably the easiest adaptation for low vision is found in the lighting aisle at your local home improvement store. Bright lighting can make a huge difference in the safety of navigating through hallways, around tables and other furnishings, as well as performing daily household and self-care tasks. Daylight bulbs are available at most places where light bulbs are sold. In addition, standing floor lamps are available with bright daylight lumens from big box stores like Walmart, Target and Lowe's as well as online stores.

It is important to place lighting strategically. Bright floor lamps should be angled away from the user's face and focused to best illuminate activities. Avoid placing lighting where it may create a reflected glare that strains the eyes. Make sure there are plenty of sources of lighting available in work areas, pathways, and higher traffic areas in the home.

Well-lit hallways and bathrooms are impor-tant during the nighttime trips to the bath-room. You can use motion sensor and touch lights to help keep your sleeping quarters dark until you need to get up to use the bathroom.

When possible, take advantage of natural lighting in your home. Control the direction of the light and decrease the glare of natural light with adjustable blinds and curtains.

IMPROVE ACCESSIBILITY WITH CONTRASTING COLOR AND TEXTURES

You can also make your home safer for the vision impaired by using textured items and contrasting colors in creative ways. Following are some ideas you can try, but as you adapt your home to your specific needs, you may find even more functional ways to make changes using the ideas here.

## Using Color for Improved Accessibility

Switch plates become easier to locate when they contrast with the wall color. You can achieve this effect with paint or brightly colored tape or switch plate covers.

Doorways will be easier to locate if you paint door frames in bright or contrasting colors.

Bright colors and textures can also be added to controls on stoves, microwaves, electronic devices, faucet handles, door knobs, drawer pulls and grab bars. Bright, contrasting paint can be added to steps and stairs to make bottom and top steps more visible. You can add sand or an anti-slip paint additive to provide added friction for fall prevention.

· · ·

As I mentioned in an earlier section, rugs in the home are discouraged. However, if you *must* use a rug in your home, use one of contrasting color to the floor, making sure it is anchored down securely. This is especially important when there is someone in the home who has impaired vision.

USING TEXTURE FOR IMPROVED ACCESSIBILITY

Cabinet bumpers, also called bump dots, are adhesive-backed shock absorbers that can be used to improve tactile navigation of keypads and remote controls. Bump dots can be found in a variety of colors at home improvement stores, office supply stores, and online. Puff paint, available in a variety of bold, bright colors, can be used for the same purpose and is available wherever craft supplies are sold.

Textured fabrics on furniture can provide tactile cues for safety and comfort when used on chairs, sofas, and beds for example. Brightly colored hand towels on armrests can help you achieve proper alignment with chairs and sofas before sitting.

These environmental strategies allow individuals to engage their tactile senses, supplementing their visual perception to support independence and safety in activities related to meal preparation, household management, and self-care.

AIDING ACCESSIBILITY WITH EQUIPMENT

We usually think of grab bars as bathroom equipment, but grab bars can also be used as navigation aids for the visually impaired. Grab bars can be mounted vertically or horizontally to mark entries and provide hand holds for moving through doorways. I've also seen stair rails used in a similar fashion, installed horizontally along the length of a hallway to provide stability and tactile cues that mark the end of the hall.

· · ·

Handrails used on staircases or steps generally extend slightly beyond the top and bottom steps for safety. For improved fall prevention with low vision, a strip of textured tape can also be placed strategically on handrails to indicate the bottom and top steps.

Nowadays there are a plethora of higher tech products available to assist individuals with low vision and hearing impairments. But the low-tech approach will go a long way to keep you and family members safe when applied strategically.

## ROUTINES AND STRATEGIES
## TO IMPROVE SAFETY

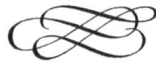

B y the time we reach a certain age, most of us have experienced a tragedy or other misfortune that disrupted our lives, causing pain and trauma for ourselves and others.

Commonly, people try to rack their brains to figure out how it could have been avoided. If only we could go back and do something—anything—differently, the outcome might have been different. If only we'd taken a different route, locked that gate, gone at a different time, fixed the windshield wipers, taken off that day, etc. When a tragedy happens, these thoughts are maddening, but normal.

My goal in this chapter is to give you strategies and encouragement to develop a proactive mindset for preventing accidents and improving safety and security in the home.

In addition to creating a safe environment in your home, there are routines, habits, and strategies that can increase your security even more. Your home will be safe not only for you but for your guests. When you go to sleep at night, you can rest well knowing you and your home are safe and secure. And just as important, your family members will know that you have a mindset that will serve to keep you safe long after other families begin to worry that mom or dad may not be safe to stay home alone. By cultivating this mindset with these routines, habits, and strategies, your life will likely be longer, your body and relationships will be stronger, and you will likely hold onto your independence much longer, maybe till the end of your life.

ROUTINES TO IMPROVE SAFETY

When I wake in the morning, the first thing I do is flip on the coffee pot. The pot is ready to brew coffee because I prepared it as part of my nightly routine. After the coffee begins to brew, I go to the bathroom, do my morning grooming, tidy up the bathroom, then return to the kitchen to pour myself a cup of coffee. I follow this routine every single morning I spend at home, whether I have to go to work or not.

My routine allows me to get the important things done in my morning without having to think about what to do next. I never have to put this stuff on a to-do list because I've done it so consistently, for so long, it's part of my life. In fact, when I go out of town to visit relatives or take a vacation, I can become very agitated in the mornings because my routine is disrupted. I find it much harder to concentrate and to locate items I need to get ready for the day. My concentration suffers because the whole morning routine has been thrown out of whack by my change in location.

Our routines help us get through the day, particular tasks, and just make life easier in general. I want to convince you that you can create routines that will make your life safer for aging in place as well.

You probably have your own morning and evening routines. Those well-established routines are an ideal place to start to bring more safety awareness into your life.

COMMUNICATION ROUTINES TO IMPROVE SAFETY

When my children were young, "Granny" the precious woman who took care of them when I worked, had a routine of calling two of her friends every single day. She, in turn, received two phone calls from other friends every single day. These women made the calls part of their daily routine to check on one another and call for help if they were unable to get in touch with someone in the chain for a given period of time. In this way, Granny's daily routine provided a safety check for her and everyone else in the chain. She didn't have to worry about forgetting to make the calls. It was such a long-ingrained behavior, it was part of who she was.

This routine had other benefits as well, such as socialization, feeling useful, and providing a meaningful activity. I use this example to illustrate how powerful routines can be in affecting the quality and safety of your own life as well as the lives of others.

You can create such a call chain in your life to alert people in the chain if you become ill or injured. I've known people who've had falls both inside and outside their homes who laid on the hard floor or ground for hours, sometimes days, before anyone found them. Keeping a phone or an emergency call button could have averted the additional serious complications they suffered after falling and brought them help sooner.

A call chain can be designed to suit each member of the chain. Each member agrees to call one or two members, once or twice a day, during a specific time frame. Nowadays smartphones are equipped with reminders and voice-activated features so you can make a call without dropping your current activity. If you should ever fall or need help, this voice-activated feature can help you call for help.

Neighbors, family members, church members, and friends make good partners for call chains. Remember that even retirees are very busy nowadays. Be sure to keep these calls short, allowing time to exchange important information while respecting the time constraints of others in the chain.

Neighbors can also keep an eye out for one another's safety by observing routines outside the home. Communicating with neighbors about your habits, and sharing emergency contacts, can also help to keep you safe. Activities like sweeping the porch, retrieving the mail or newspaper at certain times each day can be a signal to your neighbors that all is well. Two of my neighbors had this communication routine for years. When one of them left the paper on the lawn too long her trusted neighbor knew this was a signal something was wrong, and called the emergency contact.

Having routine contact with others in your community and circle of acquaintances can enhance your safety in the home as you age in place. In addition, being part of a team that looks out for the safety of others in your circle can add meaning to your own life. You and your family members will have a little less to worry about when you establish communication routines that help monitor your safety at home.

## BEDTIME ROUTINES TO IMPROVE SAFETY

Most of us rely on routines to make our lives flow more smoothly. We have a bedtime routine that consists of turning off lights, locking doors, charging cell phones, taking medicine etc. Our daytime routines help keep us focused and ensure that the vital tasks are accomplished as they are required to keep our needs met.

Routines become automatic after a while but adding a few new tasks to your routines can improve your health and safety in your home. When changing your routines, it's a good idea to use a written list until it becomes automatic, as well. If you don't already have a bedtime routine, use the example below to create one.

. . .

## Bedtime Routine

- Take medications
- Lock the doors
- Put the phone near the bed
- Put electronic devices on chargers
- Place a bottle of water on the nightstand
- Clear clutter and obstacles from pathways
- Perform night time grooming
- Wear emergency call device
- Turn on nighttime lighting on the path to the bathroom
- Use the bathroom
- Park assistive devices such as canes, walkers, or wheelchairs by the bed

## Habits to Improve Safety

If you want to improve your routines for maximum benefit, you can include new habits to your everyday life to help keep you and others in your circle safer. The strategies below are easy to add to your current activities, but they needn't be added all at once. Try adding one or two of these items at a time. When those become routine, add a couple more until you've incorporated the ones you find useful. Continue to be proactive in your attitude toward safety and adjust your routines accordingly.

- Avoid fluids after 7 pm to reduce nighttime bathroom trips
- Call members of the call chain
- Scan and pick up clutter daily to keep pathways clear
- Keep a phone and/or emergency call device with you at all times
- Keep electronic devices charged
- Use required assistive devices, such as walkers, canes, and wheelchairs consistently
- Put house and car keys in a designated location
- Keep the doors and windows locked

- Remove questionable foods from refrigerator daily
- Eat 3 balanced meals and drink adequate fluids daily
- Exercise
- Get some sunshine and fresh air daily, if possible

## PARING DOWN YOUR HOME
## FOR SAFETY

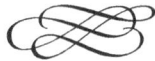

P reparing the home for aging in place involves more than just widening doorways and building ramps. Fortunately, many changes that dramatically improve safety are free.

Many people overlook how furnishings and accessories in their homes can impede safety and function. One of the simplest, but perhaps most difficult things to do to prepare your home for safely aging in place is to get rid of clutter and items that are not adding to the quality of your life. It's very important to do this task *now* while you are able, and not wait until you are literally trapped by your belongings.

I see this in my work every day. Homes become so full of furniture, books, clothing, sentimental and ornamental items, and all types of clutter individuals have collected over the years, the pathways from one room to the next and to exits, are almost impassable. These situations are depressing and difficult to live in, at best. More importantly, they present an ever-present fire and fall hazard.

Illnesses and physical deficits add to the problem and are more difficult to manage in a cluttered environment. In fact, excessive clutter and hoarding can create or contribute to physical deficits that might have otherwise been avoided had the individuals been able to deal with their belongings effectively.

. . .

Clutter can become so extreme that it becomes a literal trap, where individuals cannot move about their homes because access to living quarters, bathrooms, and exits are physically blocked. This is not an exaggeration but is a natural result of failing to address a chronic condition of too much stuff occupying too little space.

It's easy to dismiss these situations as simply messiness or unwillingness to part with sentimental items. But often the situation becomes a pathological problem where the individual is simply unable to part with their things. Family members lose patience and sometimes even abandon the individual because it may seem they don't really want help. But the individual with cluttering issues may not know how deep the problem goes or why they can't get rid of things. They just know the very thought of doing so makes them angry and extremely anxious.

.   .   .

When the problem is at this level, no amount of lecturing or even tidying up is going to deliver satisfying results. Chronic hoarding is a very common anxiety disorder and can be treated, but requires professional care.

Addressing such disorders is beyond the scope of this book, but is absolutely crucial to aging in place safely. If you believe you or your loved one has a problem with hoarding that is beyond a bit of clutter and messy habits, please seek professional help.

If you feel the clutter in your environment is just a matter of life moving faster than you can clean up the messes, then try to make decluttering a daily priority. It's a time-consuming process but is far less overwhelming if done every day. Five or ten minutes each day devoted to putting items away and sorting items to donate, put away, or throw away will create a sense of accomplishment and provide momentum to build on for the next day's session of cleaning and clearing.

Start with clearing pathways first and move to items that have been piled on surfaces that risk avalanching into the pathways. Notify community organizations such as Salvation Army and Habitat for Humanity that will pick up donations at your doorstep. Be ruthless with ridding your home of items that are compromising your safety. Remind yourself often that your safety is more important than the things you've accumulated.

Decluttering the home is every bit as impor-tant for safety as installing grab bars or en-trance ramps in the home. Books and websites abound to provide encouragement and strate-gies for clearing the clutter from your life. This is a task that is truly never done and must be addressed consistently. But the results are a happier, safer home that will support your health and safety as you age.

# CONCLUSION

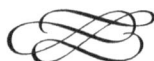

*I*t is my hope that this book has given you strategies to prevent falls and other debilitating accidents, as well as solutions to address situations that could compromise your freedom, safety, and mobility in your home as you grow older. Your home should be your haven. It should protect your health and independence. I hope this book enables you to think about your needs and to plan ahead for an active, independent life, safe in the comfort of your own home. Thank you for reading.

Lanore Dixon, COTA

# RESOURCES

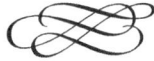

## SAFETY AND FALL PREVENTION

https://www.cdc.gov/steadi/patient.html

https://www.ncoa.org/healthy-aging/falls-prevention/falls-prevention-programs-for-older-adults-2/

https://www.cdc.gov/features/falls-prevention-day/index.html

https://www.cdc.gov/

homeandrecreationalsafety/
falls/adultfalls.html

https://www.cdc.gov/injury/features/older-
adult-falls/index.html

https://www.cdc.gov/
homeandrecreationalsafety/
falls/adultfalls.html

AGING IN PLACE AND ACCESSIBILITY RE-
SOURCES

https://www.aarp.org/livable-communities/
info-2014/aarp-home-fit-guide-aging-in-
place.html

https://www.nahb.org/Education-and-
Events/Education/Designations/Certified-
Aging-in-Place-Specialist-CAPS/Additional-
Resources/Aging-In-Place-Remodeling-
Checklist

https://www.aarp.org/states/

https://www.ada.gov/regs2010/
2010ADAStandards/2010ADAstandards.htm

AGING IN PLACE PROFESSIONALS

https://www.nahb.org/NAHB-Community/
Directories/Local-
Associations#sort=relevancy

https://www.nahb.org/Education-and-
Events/Education/Designations/Certified-
Aging-in-Place-Specialist-CAPS/Additional-
Resources/What-is-Design-for-Independent-
Living

https://homemods.org/national-directory/

https://www.aarp.org/money/scams-fraud/?
migration=rdrct

COMMUNITY AGENCIES FOR ACCESSIBILITY AS-
SISTANCE

https://www.unitedway.org/local/united-states/

https://www.habitat.org/volunteer/near-you/find-your-local-habitat

## ABOUT THE AUTHOR

As an occupational therapy practitioner, Lanore Dixon, COTA has helped thousands of individuals protect their health and independence by providing strategies to prepare themselves and their homes for successful aging in place. With her experience, readers can invest in the right equipment and strategies for safety and fall prevention to protect their independence as they prepare to age in place for the rest of their lives.

Lanore lives in Texas with her husband, two dogs, and her best friend, Rhonda. Every day provides a new opportunity to prepare the members of her household to live happily and safely ever after in their own home.

This is Lanore's first book of non-fiction.

www.ingramcontent.com/pod-product-compliance
Lightning Source LLC
Chambersburg PA
CBHW032114280326
41933CB00009B/833